TRACE IT to ERASE IT

Tap into BRAINPOWER to be happy and healthy.

Dr. Selena E. Bartlett

Neuroscientist

This book is dedicated to James and Ella. "Find your spirit and free your mind".

Books are available at special quantity discounts to corporations, schools, literacy programs, other organizations, and other large orders, please contact: info@smashmindset.com.

ISBN: 978-0-9990-9972-8

Printed in the U.S.A. and Australia.

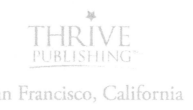

THRIVE
PUBLISHING

San Francisco, California

Trace It to be Happy and Healthy

There is nothing more forceful or powerful than BRAINPOWER.

Dr. Selena Bartlett is a neuroscientist that created an easy to follow guidebook that uses tracing and other fun techniques to help you learn how to tap into brainpower. The simple act of tracing instead of reacting to the situation helps to retrain the brain to manage stress, overcome negative thought patterns, break free of old habits, to be more positive, healthier and happier. Tracing on top of the lines, slowly and precisely, puts a pause on the emotional part of the brain, or what she calls MiGGi. You may not be able to control stress, BUT, you can control how the brain handles stress.

The brain is stronger and more resilient than you think as soon as you learn to tap into brainpower using the principles of neuroplasticity. Learn more about how to tap into brainpower to be happy and healthy at www.selenab.com.

A smile might just change someone's life.

We mirror the people that surround us. Try to find the good reflectors.

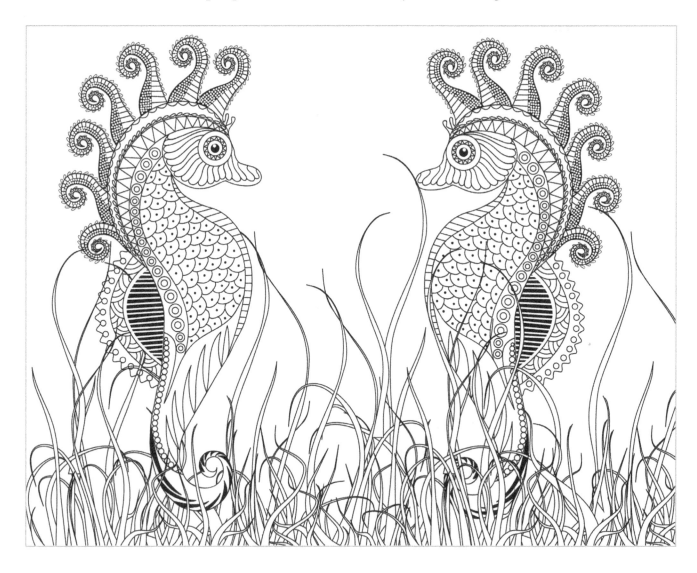

Trace It to Erase It

Step 1. Trace It. Take a fine-point pen.

Step 2. Start on any line in the picture.

Step 3. Slowly draw on top of the lines as precisely as possible.

Step 4. Take as little or as much time as needed.

Step 5. Erase It. Repeat steps 1-4 each day because practice makes perfect.

Step 6. Learn more about MiGGi or the emotional part of the brain.

Step 7. Set the brain in the right direction from the moment you wake in the morning.

Have fun on your new path to a smashing mindset.

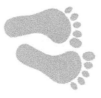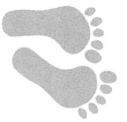

KEY TAKEAWAY:

It is not about WILLPOWER.
It is about BRAINPOWER.

Trace It to Erase It is a simple way to tap into brainpower. When you stop and trace instead of reacting to stress or an emotional situation, you are pausing the brain. This gives the brain a break and the time it needs to respond to, instead of react to, stress or the situation.

The daily and repeated practice trains the brain to learn a new way to respond to the same situation. Trace It calms the emotional part of the brain, or MiGGi, and strengthens the rational part of the brain or Thinker.

Trace on the lines slowly and precisely.

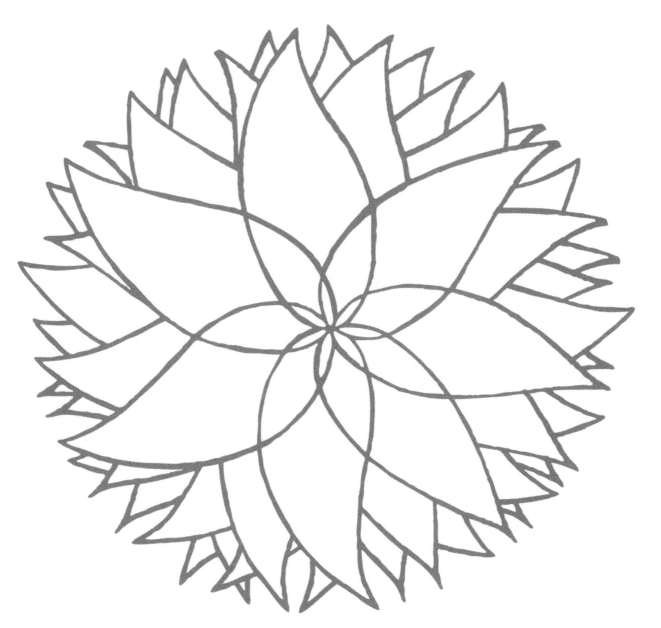

Reboot your brain.

KEY TAKEAWAY:

**Stop your brain, for one second,
to give it time to respond and not react.**

Just as, with effort and practice, the brain can learn a new language or skill, it can be changed in the way it reacts to stress or emotional situations. With repeated and daily practice tracing erases the way we react to stress. It calms the emotional part of the brain, MiGGi, and allows the rational part of the brain, or Thinker, time to respond to, instead of react to, the situation.

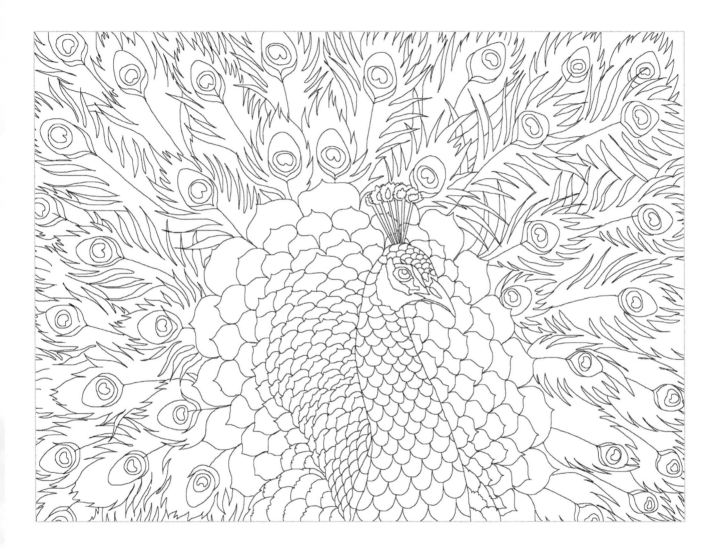

Stand tall, push your shoulders back, and know your brain is stronger than you think it is.

KEY TAKEAWAY:

Change your future stress responses by changing your brain.

It starts by teaching the brain a new trick. Trace it instead of react to it. Because MiGGi, or the emotional part of the brain, prioritizes fear and stress over love and happiness. It takes daily and repeated practice over time to rewire MiGGi for love and happiness over fear and stress.

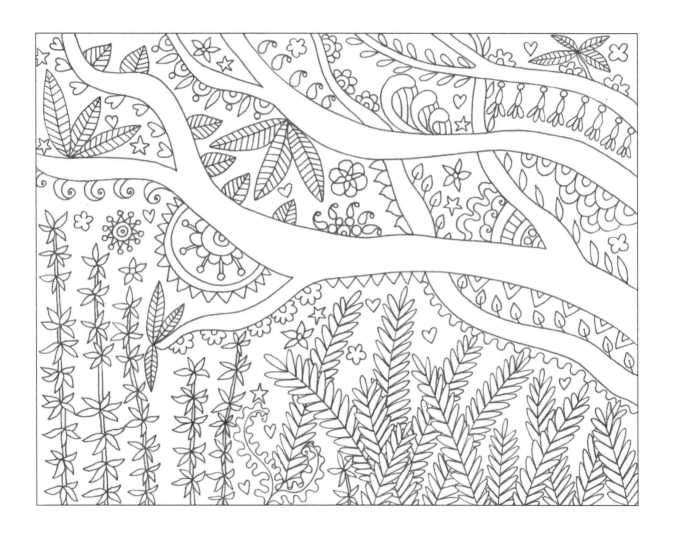

Plant the seeds, grow your mindset.

Smile.

Love in all its forms energizes the brain, and fills it with feel-good chemicals, like endorphins and oxytocin. This is why a smile, a hug, or a simple touch feels wonderful. Every brain has an unlimited capacity for love. You can train the brain to love.

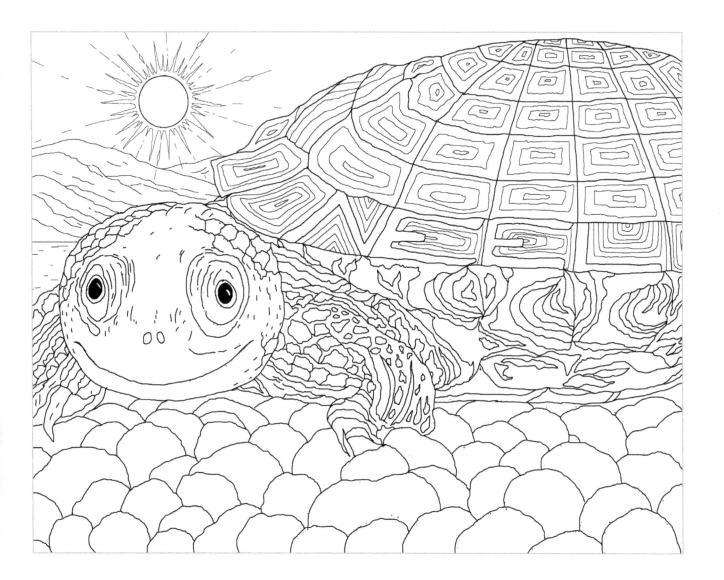

Love is viral and radiates onwards.

KEY TAKEAWAY:

**Simply put, if you don't handle stress,
the brain finds a way to handle it for you.**

Become more aware of your stress reactions or MiGGi moments. That is, when the emotional part of the brain is over-riding the rational part of the brain. If you are stressed or worried try tracing instead.

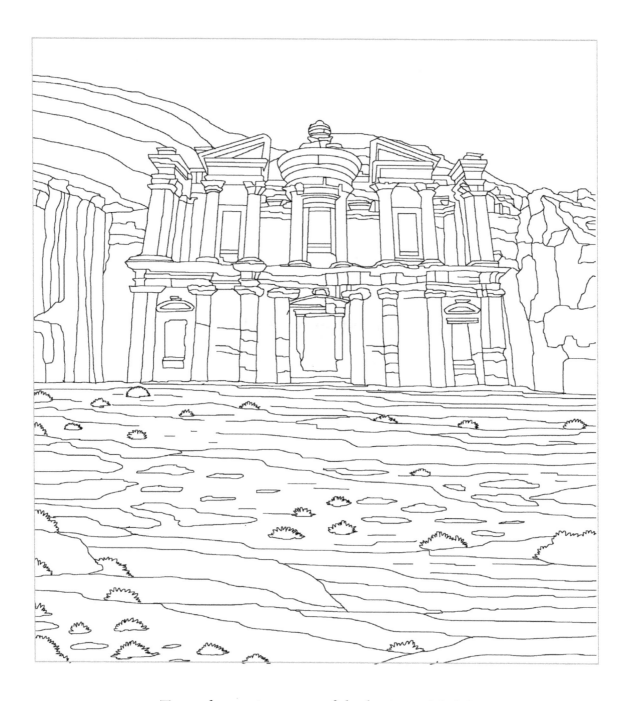

Tame the ancient part of the brain or MiGGi.

KEY TAKEAWAY:

Breathe, Stop and Think.

Breathe in through your nose for four seconds, then breathe out through your mouth for four seconds. Breathing calms MiGGi for a second and this allows the brain enough time to engage Thinker.

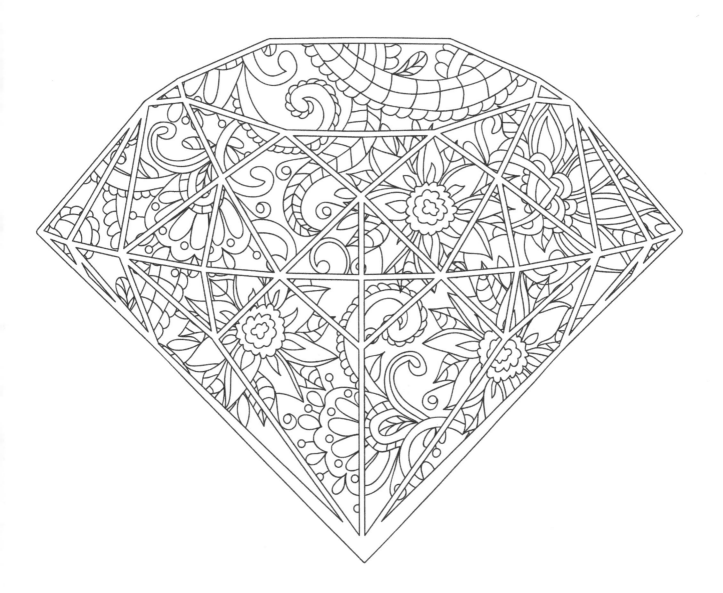

A shiny diamond lies inside MiGGi waiting to be polished.

KEY TAKEAWAY:

Pause MiGGi to activate Thinker.

MiGGi is the emotional part of the brain that reacts to stress in milliseconds, often before you are aware of it. Tracing helps to pause MiGGi to enable enough time to engage the rational part of the brain or Thinker. This allows the brain enough time to respond in a calmer and more rational way. When MiGGi reacts it tends to rely on gut instincts and pulls out strategies it learnt from the distant past to solve stressful situations. The majority of the time, MiGGi reactions tend to be less than optimal solutions to the problem at hand compared to Thinker responses.

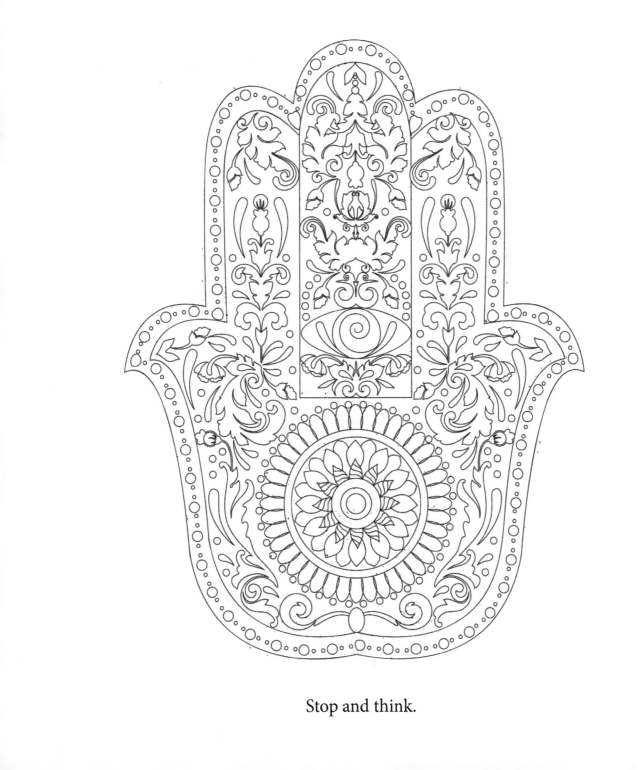

Stop and think.

The brain is stronger than you think.

The brain has an amazing and untapped potential for change using the principles of neuroplasticity. The key is to learn how to unlock MiGGi reactions and turn them into Thinker responses. This is because stress locks up the brain and keeps it stuck in an unending loop. When you train the brain, by taking a daily brain break, you have tapped into brainpower. Tracing is a simple way to get started.

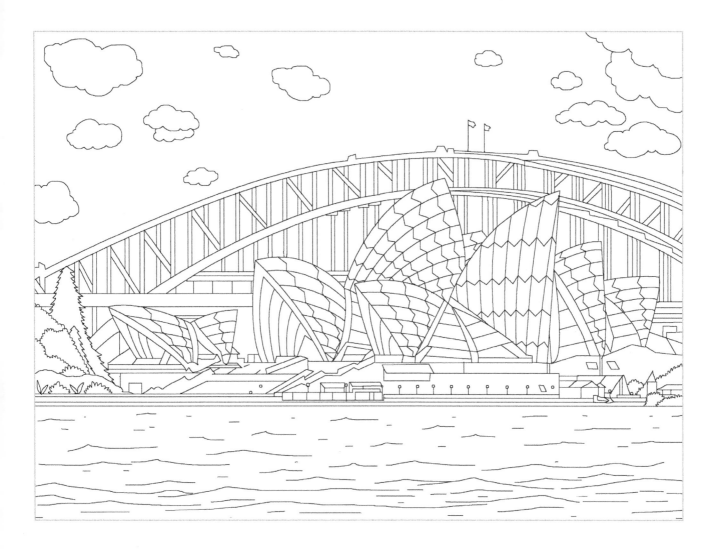

You can make your dreams happen.

KEY TAKEAWAY:

Push your shoulders back. Take a deep breath. Trace.

It has been shown that your body posture affects both the stress and power hormone levels in your body. When you push your shoulders back and take a deep breath, the stress hormone cortisol is lower and the power hormone testosterone is higher. Try this before something stressful, like a difficult conversation, an interview, a test or going on a date. This improves your confidence and presence.

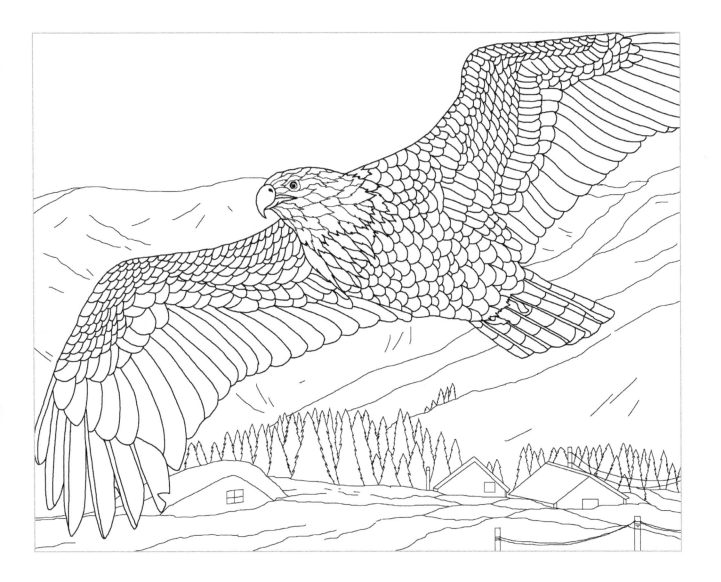

Train your brain. Free your brain.

KEY TAKEAWAY:

The brain needs a detox too.

The brain is like a learning machine. The more we think about something, good or bad, the more the brain will find a way to make it happen for you. Train the brain to stop going over the past. Nothing can be changed, except what we do in this second and at this moment. Train the brain everyday to focus on this moment and positive things and see what unfolds.

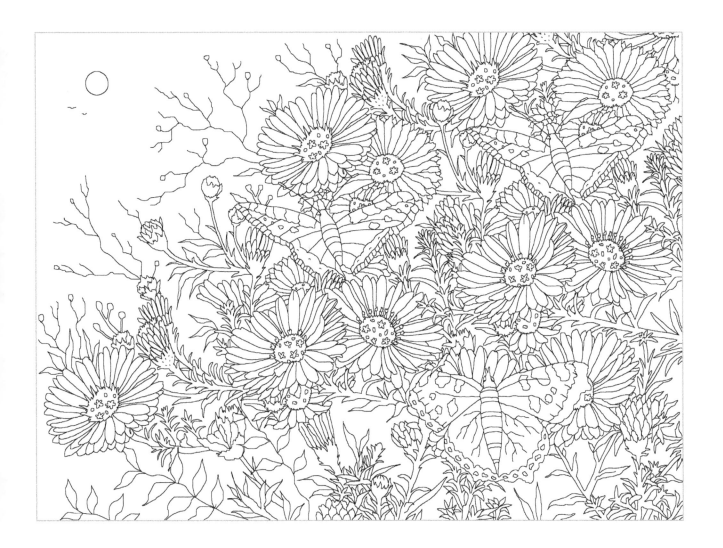

Give the brain a spring clean.

KEY TAKEAWAY:

Let It Go!

Write here what was going through your mind while tracing then let it go. This is a way to train the ancient part of the brain or (MiGGi) to not react. The repeated practice turns MiGGi reactions to Thinker responses. Then you learn a new way to respond to stressful or emotional situations.

_____

_____

_____

_____

_____

_____

_____

_____

_____

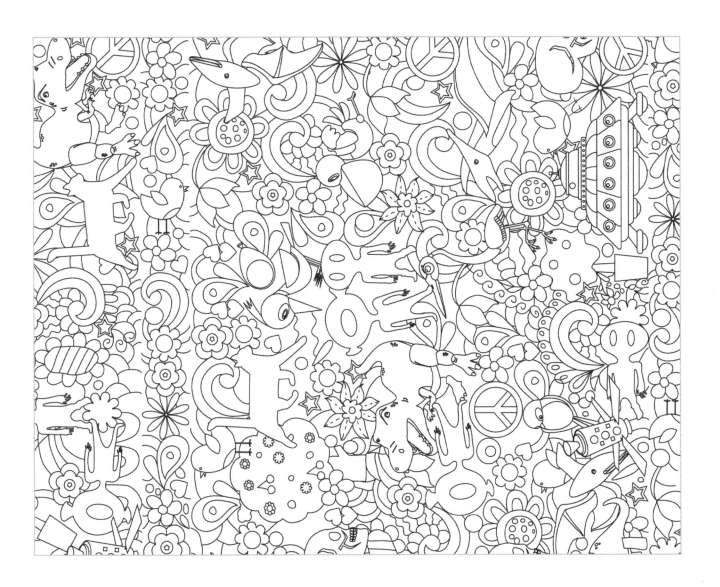

Unlock the beauty trapped inside the ancient part of the brain or MiGGi.

KEY TAKEAWAY:

Draw a line in the sand and step forward.

The brain likes to hold onto old solutions to solve problems, as a way to make us feel safe. That is, we think we know how to fix any problem or stress we face. When the brain was young, it learnt how to solve stressful situations or problems and was very clever at finding great solutions. These solutions have kept you alive. However, sometimes a young brain's solutions to MiGGi reactions do not always work as you grow and change over time. This is why we have to draw a line in the sand to the past, and move forward by training the brain to solve MiGGi reactions in grown up ways.

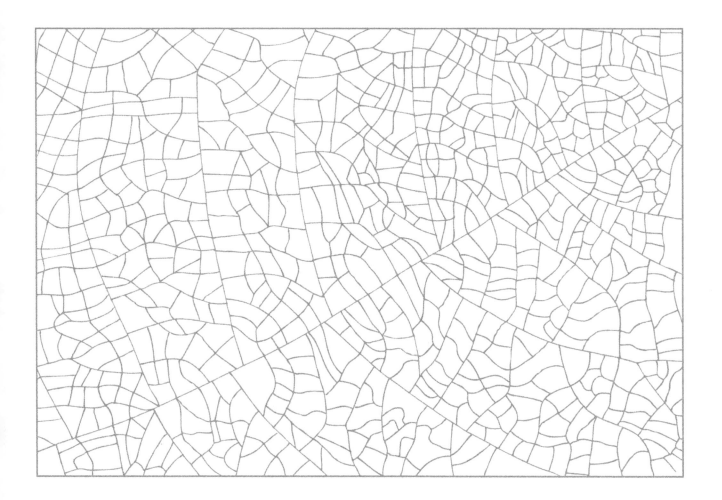

Sprout new brain connections.

KEY TAKEAWAY:

Smile

Smiling promotes feel-good chemicals like endorphins and dopamine. Try smiling at another person and see them smile back.

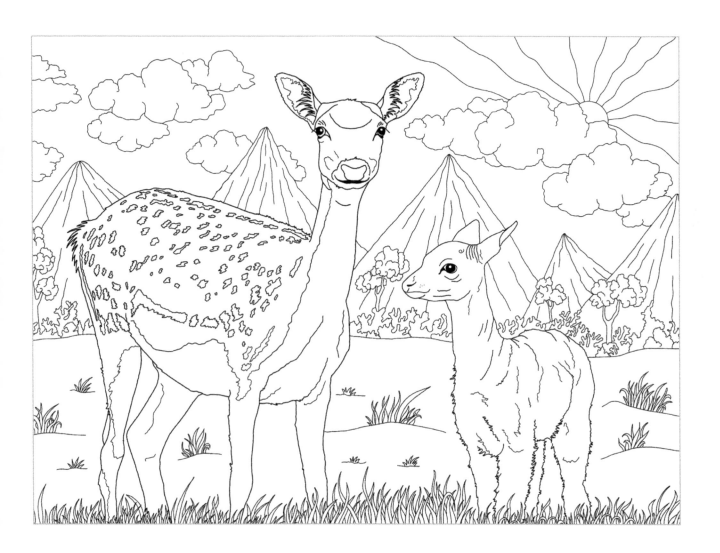

Everyone loves a smile.

KEY TAKEAWAY:

Every brain deserves a good start.

Try kick starting your brain by looking into the beauty of nature.

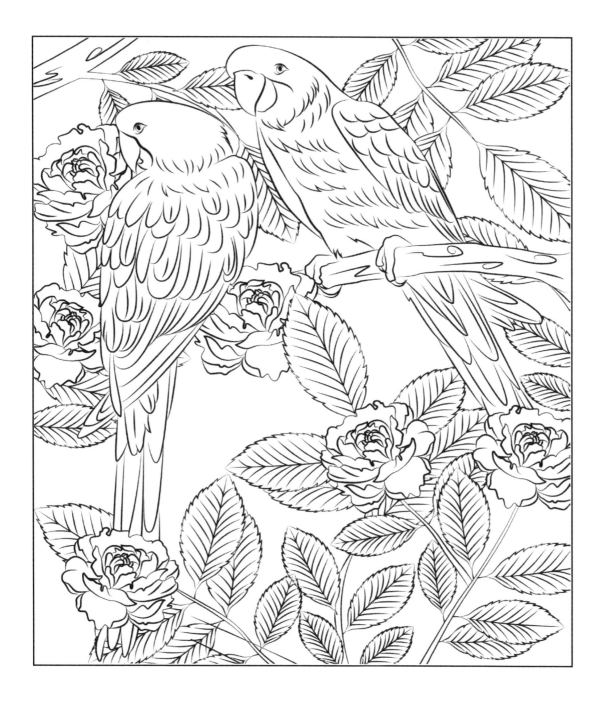

The essence radiating out from nature calms the brain.

KEY TAKEAWAY:

Stop MiGGi moments by doing something else instead.

Stress locks down the brain and makes it hard to change. Start to notice when stress triggers the emotional part of your brain and then ask yourself "Am I having a MiGGi moment? When you notice MiGGi moments on a daily basis you become more aware of them. Then you can learn how to stop MiGGi moments in their tracks. The best way is to do something else instead. Like take a deep breath or trace.

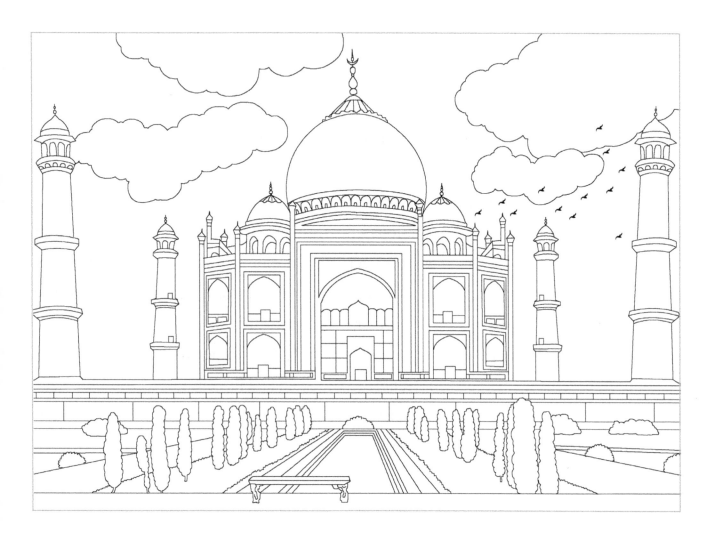

The brain is magnificent and begs to be trained.
Train the brain like you train the muscles in your body.

KEY TAKEAWAY:

Stop MiGGi moments in their tracks.

You can change the way your brains work using the principles of neuroplasticity, that is training the brain to turn MiGGi reactions into Thinker responses. Start to pay attention to MiGGi moments. Ask yourself what triggers my emotional brain to react. For the next 28 days, train the brain to stop a MiGGi moment by doing something else instead. For example, instead of having a MiGGi moment, and throwing the saucepan, eating a tub of ice-cream or a block of chocolate, trace it. Train MiGGi to not react and let Thinker respond. By practising this, you can strengthen the brain and its communication channels. Eventually, MiGGi and Thinker learn a new form of communication. This is how you turn a MiGGi moment into a Thinker response.

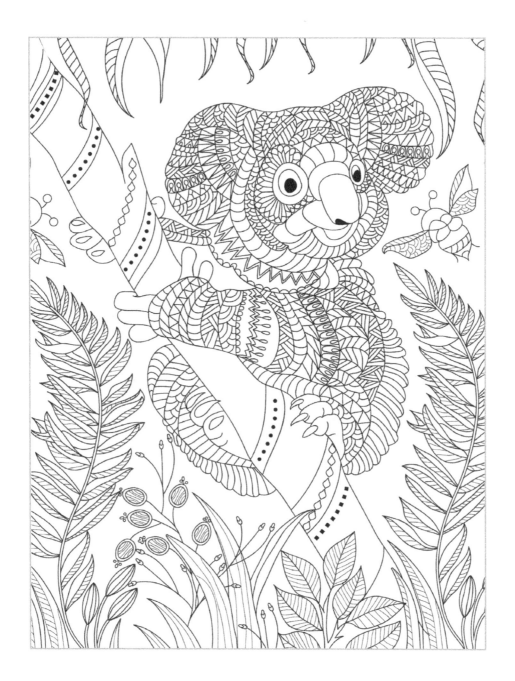

Get into Thinker mode.

KEY TAKEAWAY:

Balance stress with healthy rewards.

The brain needs to get feel-good chemicals to counter-balance the toxic effects of chemicals from over-reacting to worry and stress. Tracing is a healthy way to promote feel-good brain chemicals in response to stressful situations.

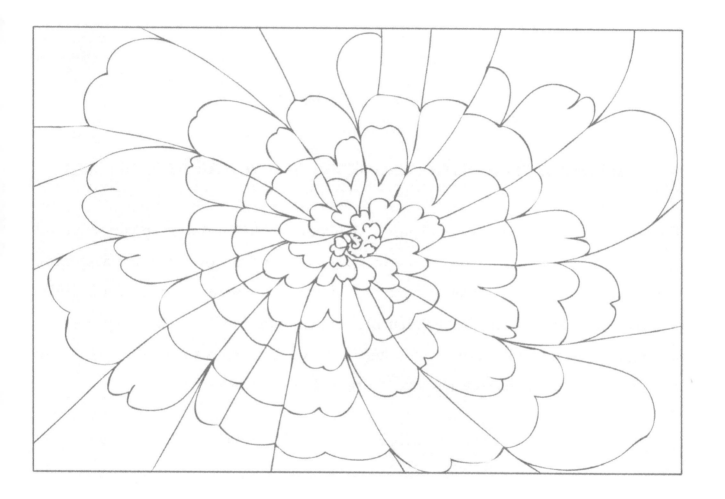

Pollinate the brain with feel-good chemicals like dopamine and oxytocin.

KEY TAKEAWAY:

The brain prefers fear and stress to love and happiness.

The main purpose of the emotional part of the brain or MiGGi is to keep you safe from physical threats. This is why the brain prioritizes stress and fear over love and happiness. When you put the little stresses and worries on replay, the brain learns that it is under constant threat and this can become harmful to the brain. MiGGi is balancing stress by seeking rewards in the form of alcohol, sugar, or food. Tracing is a healthier way to give the brain a reward and learn a new way to respond to stress or worry.

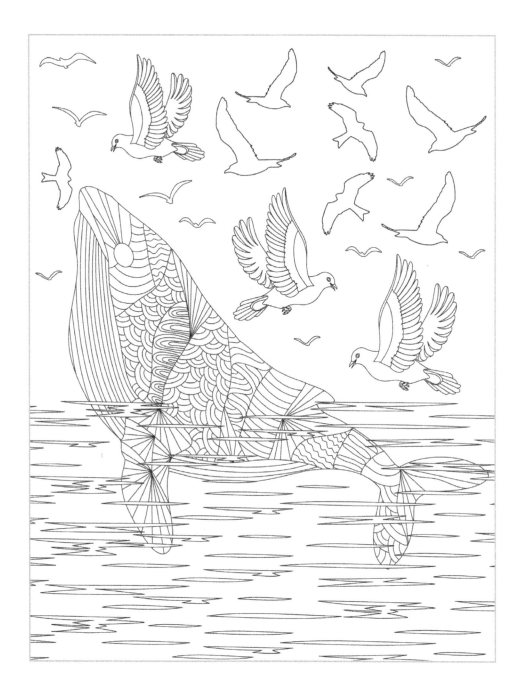

Train MiGGi to seek healthy rewards.

KEY TAKEAWAY:

Trace It instead of Eat and/or Drink It.

For example, after a stressful day at work or school, you may go to the fridge or vending machine and have ice-cream, chocolate, a sugary drink, or eat a packet of chips. Instead of over-eating when you are stressed out, try tracing instead.

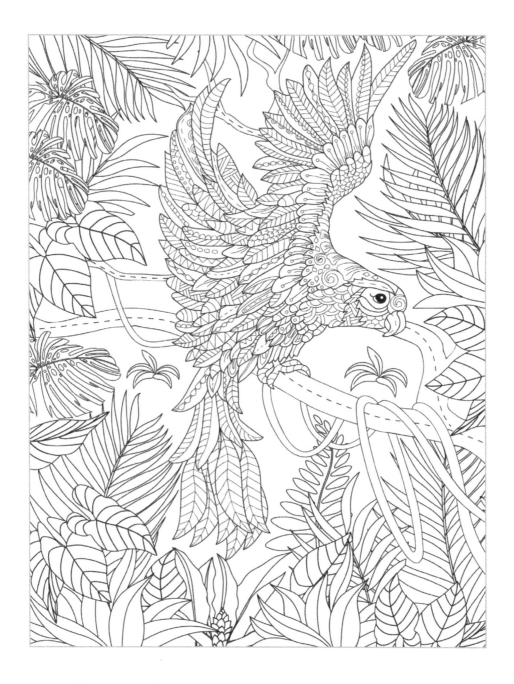

It all starts with setting the brain in a good direction every morning. Hit the reset button as soon as you wake.

Trace It to Move It.

Dopamine is a brain chemical that gets you to move, feel pleasure and motivated. If you are stressed and reach for a bag of chips; this gives the brain a quick pleasure fix and relieves stress for the moment. Instead try to train the brain to seek dopamine from healthier habits, like tracing or going for a walk. You have learnt a way to manage stress for a lifetime.

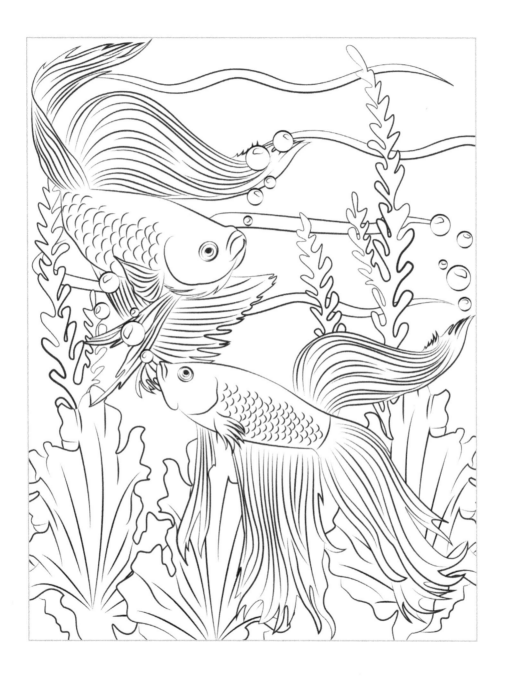

Give a person a fish and they eat for a day,
teach them how to fish and they eat for a lifetime.

KEY TAKEAWAY:

Love is without bounds. Hate has an ending.

The brain has an unlimited capacity for love. The brain can be trained to love more. The love supply is only limited by stress, fear and when we cut it off. Love sprays the brain with protective chemicals from the day the brain started developing. Unconditional love heals nearly all wounds.

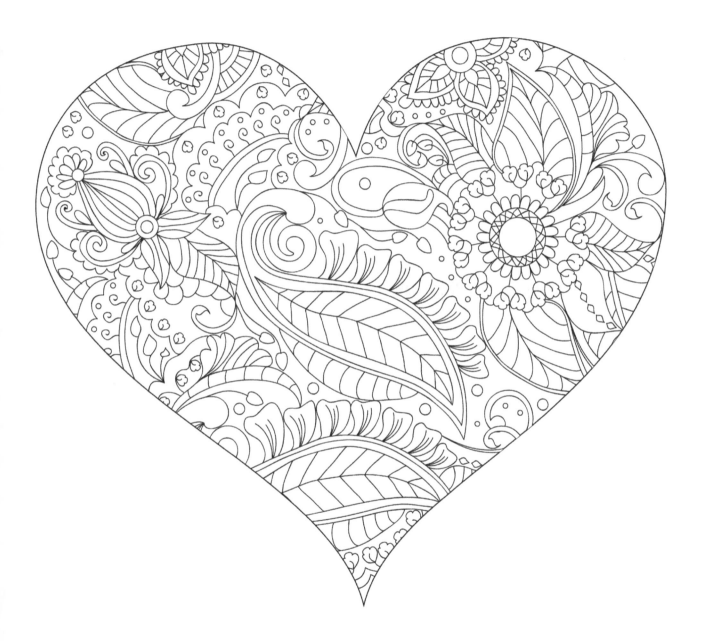

Love is an antidote to stress.

KEY TAKEAWAY:

Stress leaves an imprint in our bodies.

The brain balances stress with rewards like sugar, alcohol, high fat foods and beverages. The excess energy from these type of foods and beverages is stored in the fat cells in our tummies and thighs.

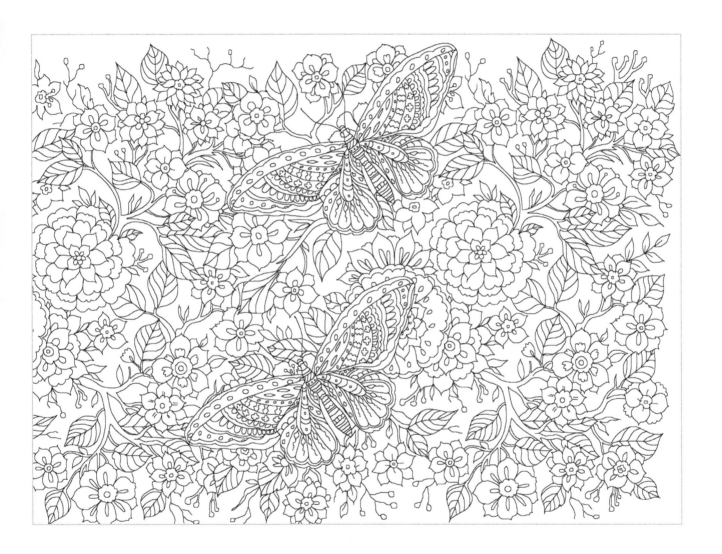

Connect with nature to stop MiGGi moments.

KEY TAKEAWAY:

Train the brain to prioritize happiness over stress.

Unfortunately for some of us, MiGGi or the emotional part of the brain is hard-wired for fear, stress, and pain more than pleasure or happiness. That's because the brain's main goal is our survival. The good news is, we can train the brain to do the opposite. Prioritize happiness over stress. Tracing is a great way to start!

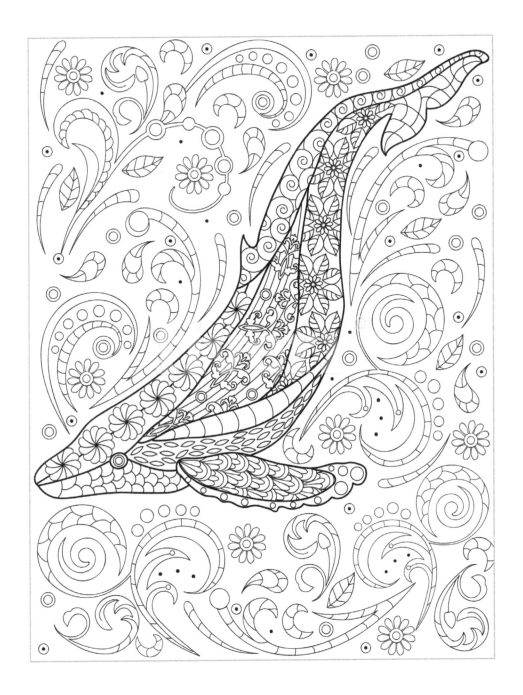

Try to choose your good side.

KEY TAKEAWAY:

Exercise stops MiGGi so you can think.

Exercise has been shown to reduce stress responses and inflammation. Exercise increases the expression of genes that promote brain plasticity, including the generation of new neurons and blood vessels. Start by standing instead of sitting, or move your arms.

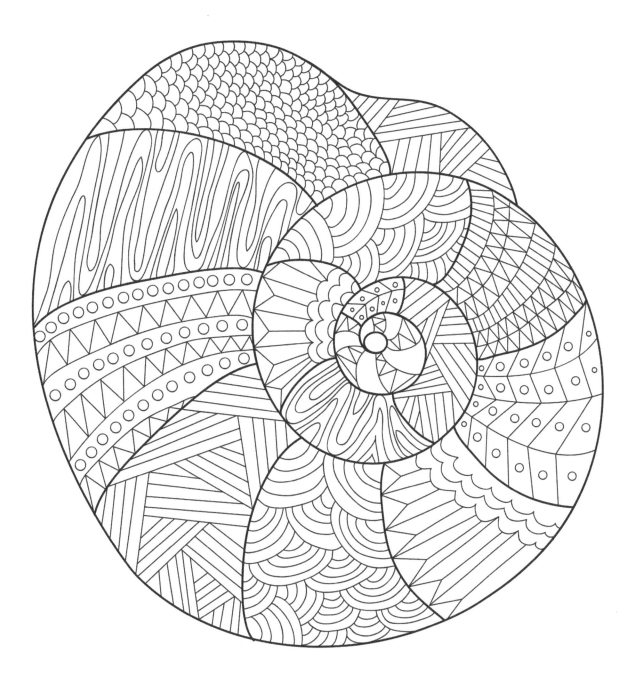

Spiral up and out of the emotional part of the brain or MiGGi.

KEY TAKEAWAY:

Too much sugar makes us feel more stressed.

Fructose in sugar activates the emotional part of our brain or MiGGi and makes you feel more stressed. The energy from excess fructose is stored in the visceral fat cells. The ones in tummies and at the top of our thighs. Don't quit eating sugar all at once, but slowly reduce the amount you eat.

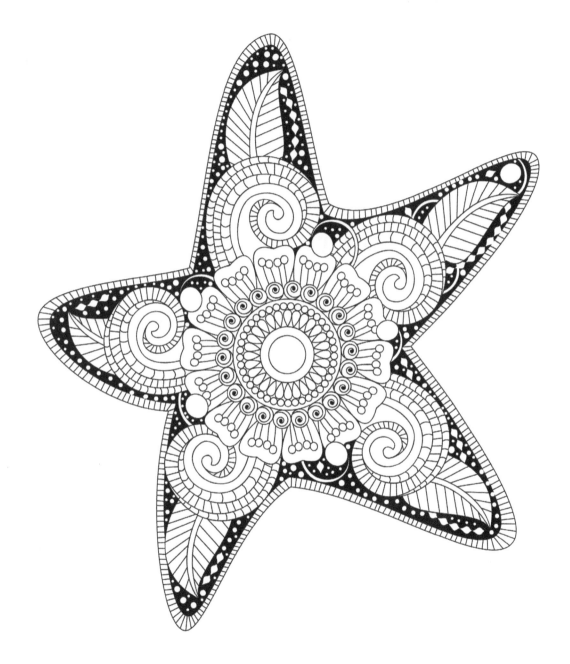

Reset mindset. Grow brainpower.

KEY TAKEAWAY:

Get the oxytocin rush by tracing with friends.

Oxytocin is the chemical needed for bonding and love. Tracing with friends keeps us connected and our brain happy and healthy.

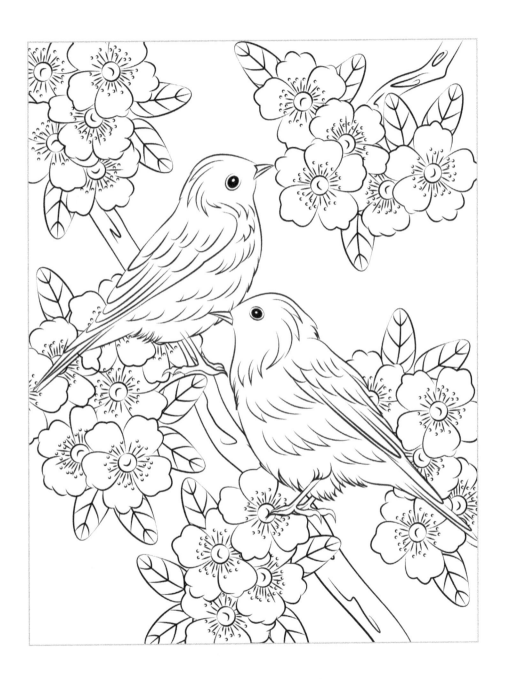

Connections matter more than stress.

KEY TAKEAWAY:

Let It Go!

Write here what was going through your mind while tracing then let it go. This is a way to train the ancient part of the brain or (MiGGi) to not react. The repeated practice turns MiGGi reactions to Thinker responses. Then you learn a new way to respond to stressful or emotional situations.

_____

_____

_____

_____

_____

_____

_____

_____

_____

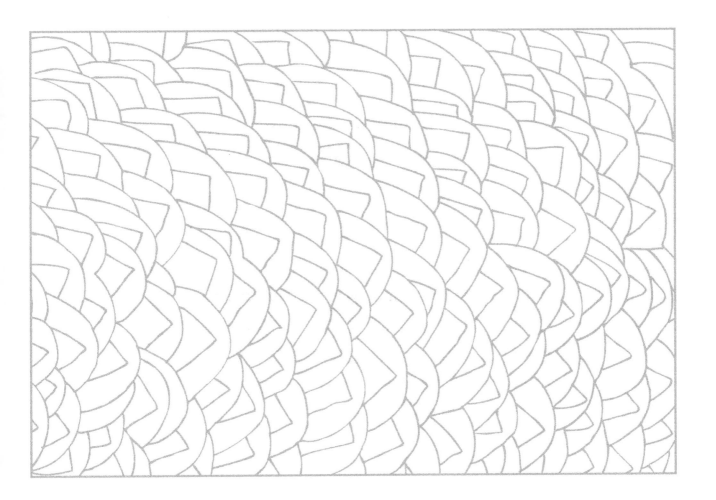

Be more compassionate to your brain and how clever it is.

KEY TAKEAWAY:

Smile

Smiling activates mirror neurons. Try smiling at another person and they will smile back at you.

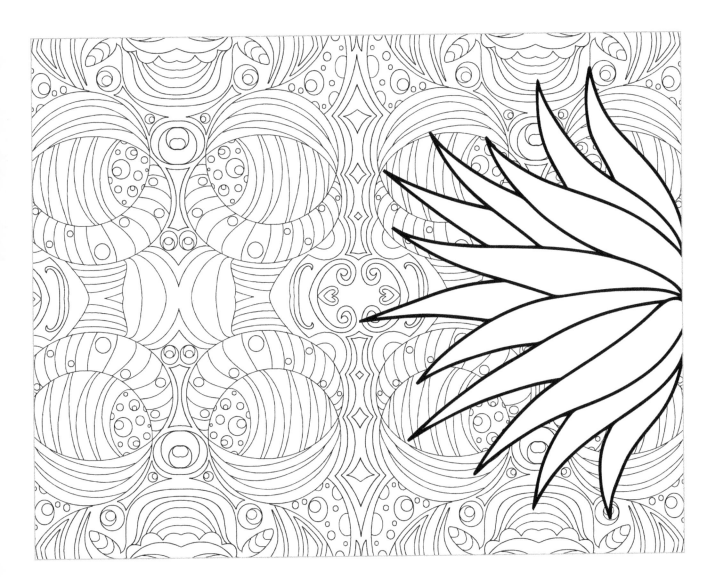

Give some positive vibes to others.

KEY TAKEAWAY:

Stand instead of sit to trace.

Sitting for more than six hours a day makes us less trim and unhealthy.

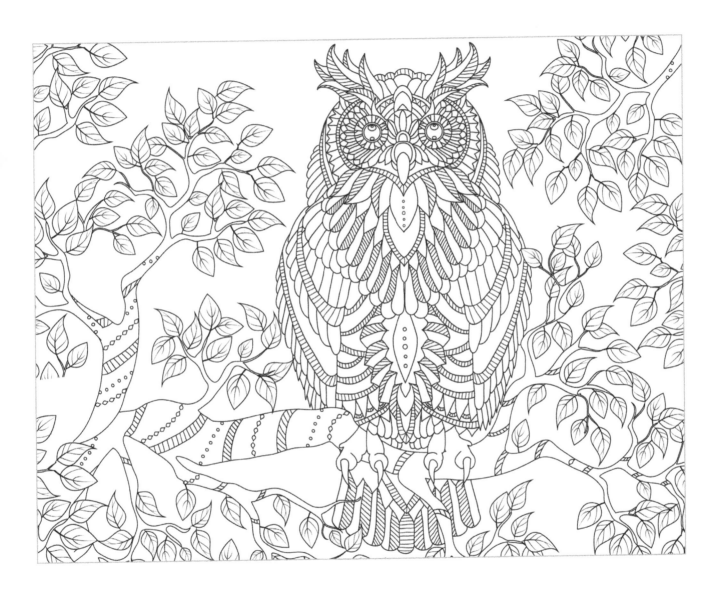

Exercise grows the brain.

KEY TAKEAWAY:

Embrace joy.

Every morning when you wake embrace the beauty not the beast.

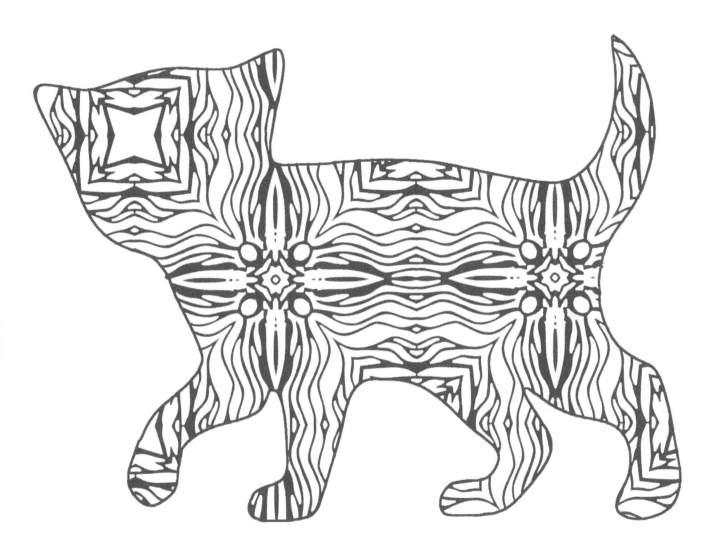

Pause for a second and accept the happiness radiating toward you.

KEY TAKEAWAY:

We have to get up and move!

Tracing is a great way to clear the brain and get motivated. Otherwise we have to do 60-75 mins of exercise everyday to counter the effects of sitting for long periods of time.

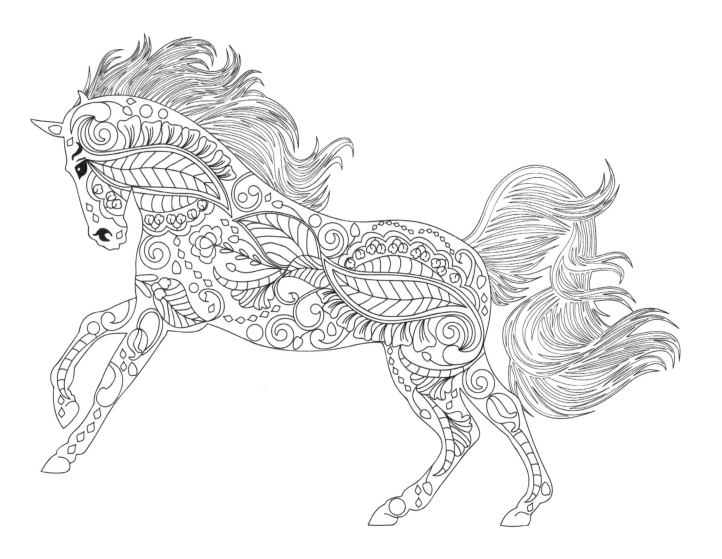

Get back up and recharge your body.

KEY TAKEAWAY:

Love is the antidote to stress.

Love in all its glory ignites the beautiful chemicals in the brain. What a perfect way to counter-balance the stress chemicals. Reach out and call, send a note of encouragement, touch someone that matters to you.

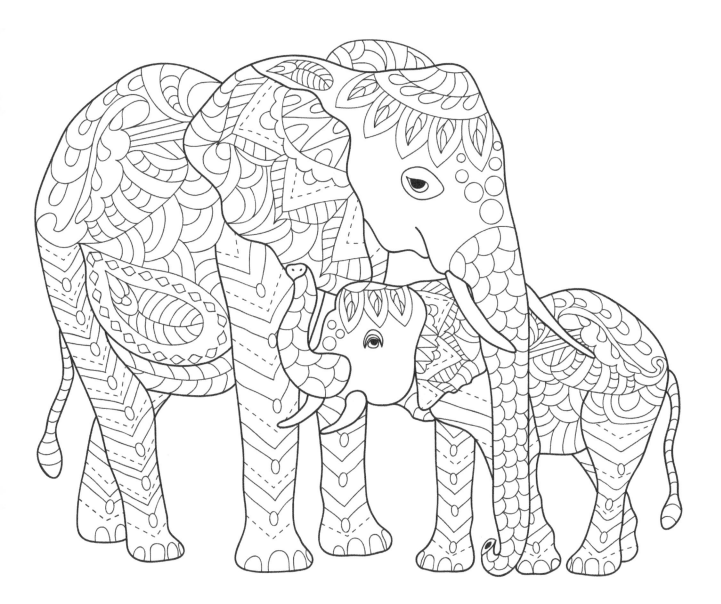

Make love go viral.

KEY TAKEAWAY:

Pause MiGGi to activate Thinker.

MiGGi is the emotional part of the brain that reacts to stress in milliseconds, often before we are aware of it. We have to use tools to pause it long enough to engage thinker.

Tracing helps to pause MiGGi and give the brain time to engage the rational part of the brain to respond more thoughtfully to an emotional situation.

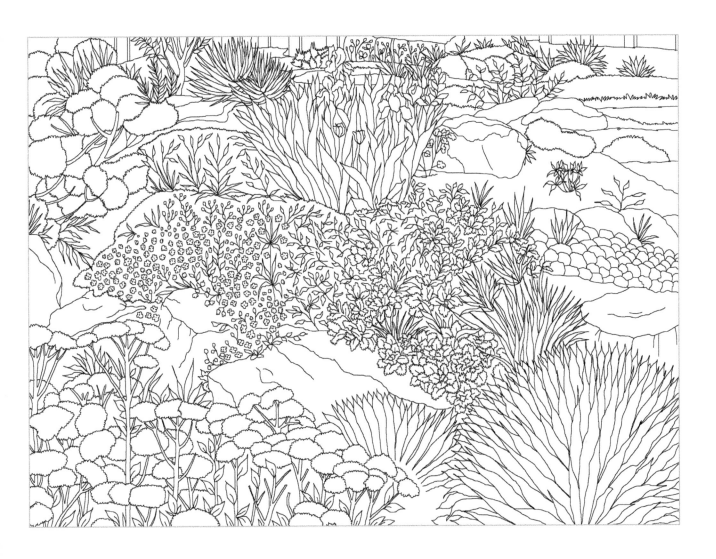

Prioritize nature over stress.

KEY TAKEAWAY:

Train the brain using the power of neuroplasticity and epigenetics.

The brain is governed by an inherited genetic code (genetics) and over time the brain is shaped by the environment and experiences (epigenetics). While everyone's brain is capable of change, by applying the principles of neuroplasticity and taking daily actions, each of us have experienced varying amounts of stress during our lives. Stress wires the brain and this is why it is takes longer for some people to train MiGGi than for others.

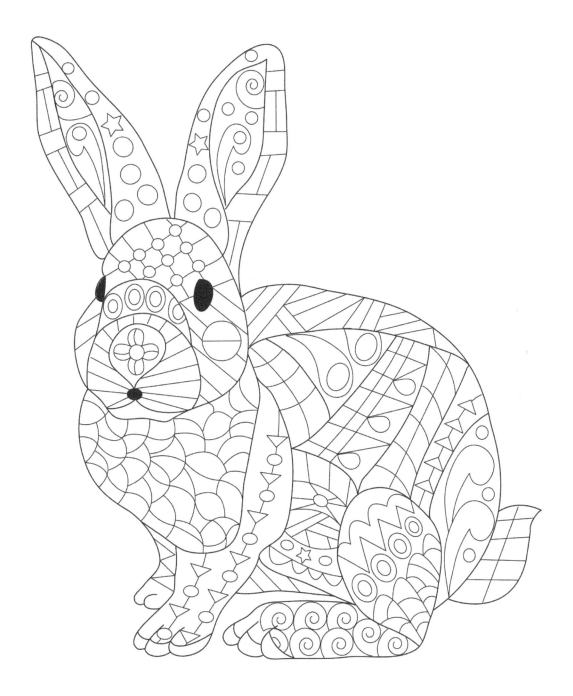

Neuroplasticity is the magic that unlocks brainpower.

KEY TAKEAWAY:

Put good thoughts on repeat not bad thoughts.

The brain learns by repetition. We have to pay attention to what we are repeating to ourselves.

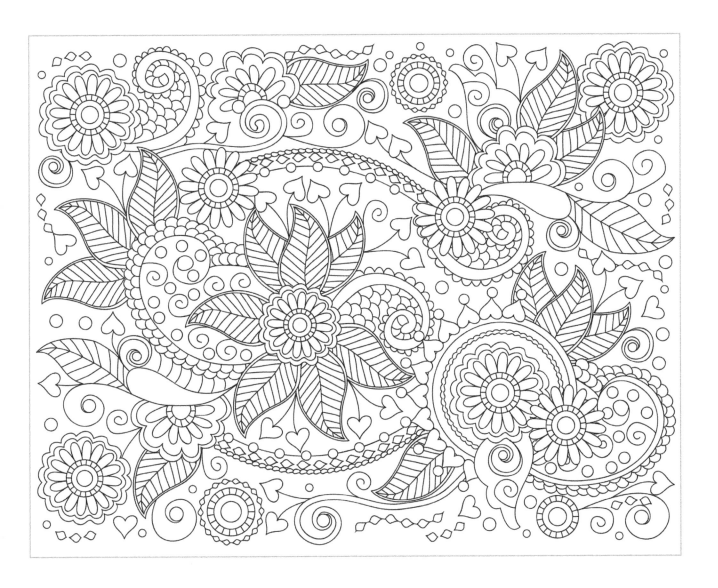

Create a happy brain by surrounding yourself with happy people and a healthy environment.

KEY TAKEAWAY:

Trace It to Waist It.

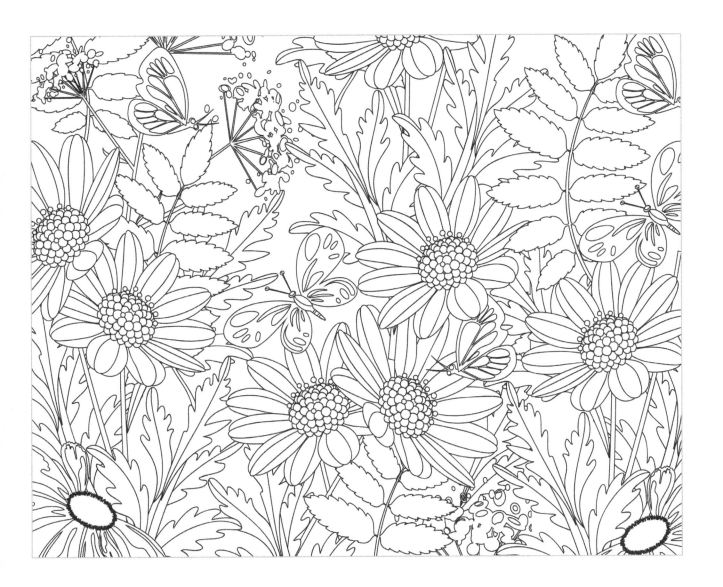

Every morning offers a new page to rewrite your brain story.

KEY TAKEAWAY:

Let It Go!

Write here what was going through your mind while tracing then let it go. This is a way to train the ancient part of the brain or (MiGGi) to not react. The repeated practice turns MiGGi reactions to Thinker responses. Then you learn a new way to respond to stressful or emotional situations.

_____

_____

_____

_____

_____

_____

_____

_____

_____

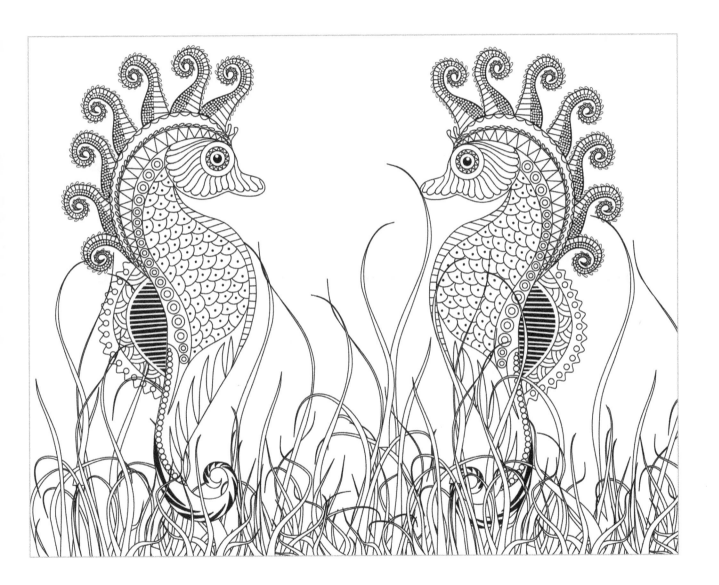

We mirror the people that surround us. Try to find the good reflectors.

When we do not manage stress then stress manages us.

Tracing calms MiGGi and strengthens Thinker. Practice letting go of the things you cannot change.

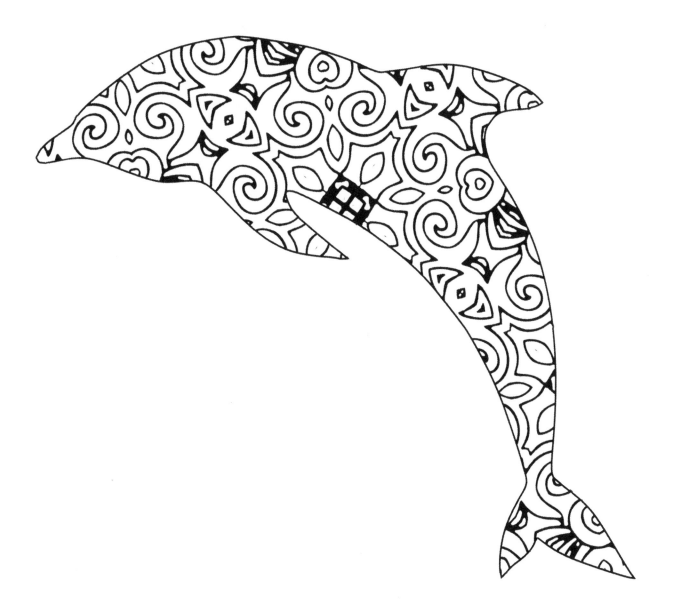

Let it all go.
Let your brain be free of the things it cannot change.

KEY TAKEAWAY:

Push your shoulders back.
Take a deep breath.
Trace It.

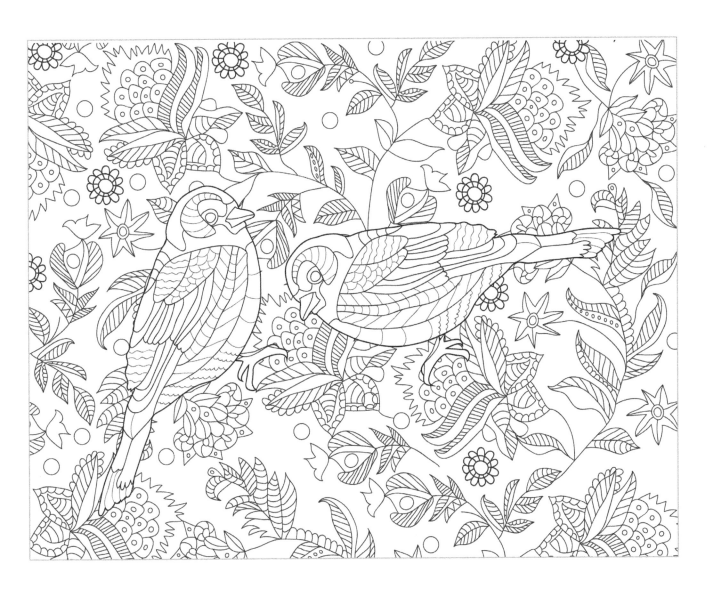

Stop, look up and pay attention to the beauty that surrounds us.

You have got this!

Smash your old mindset and reboot your brain.

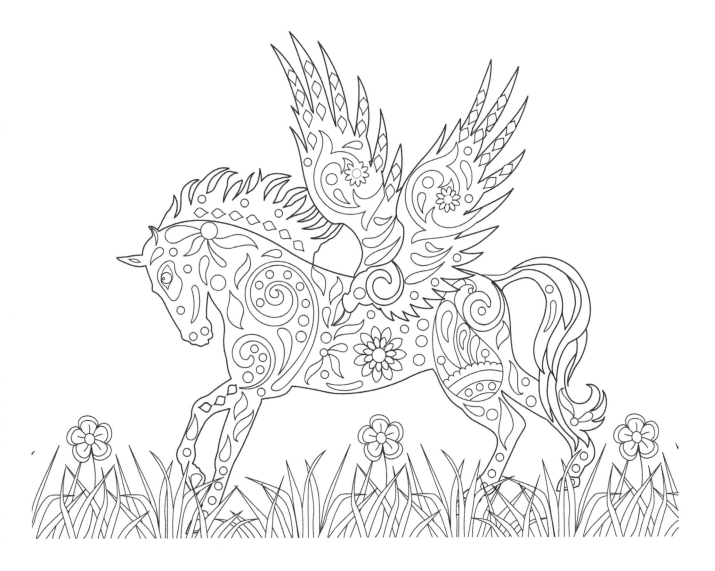

Train your brain, lift your wings, free your mind.

KEY TAKEAWAY:

Let It Go!

Write here what was going through your mind while tracing then let it go. This is a way to train the ancient part of the brain or (MiGGi) to not react. The repeated practice turns MiGGi reactions to Thinker responses. Then you learn a new way to respond to stressful or emotional situations.

_____

_____

_____

_____

_____

_____

_____

_____

_____

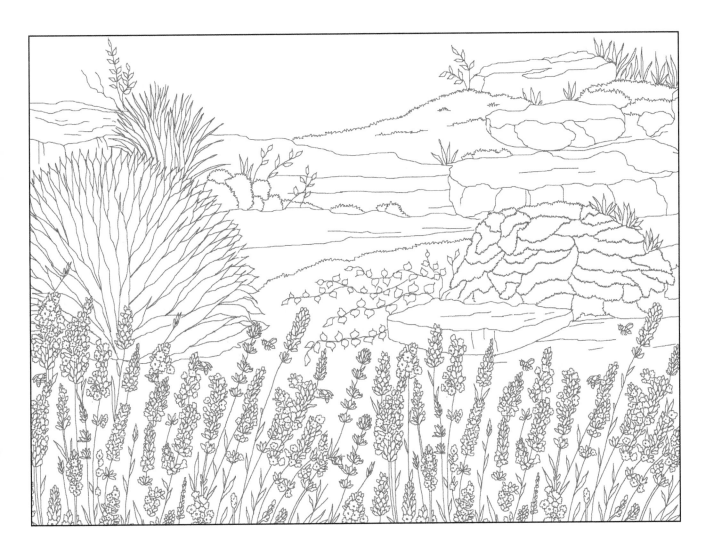

Train your brain to free your mind.

KEY TAKEAWAY:

Every brain, no matter what age, is capable of change.

Every brain has been wired differently from a life time of stress and has the capacity to change with enough effort and practice. Tracing trains the brain to calm MiGGi and strengthen Thinker or the rational part of the brain.

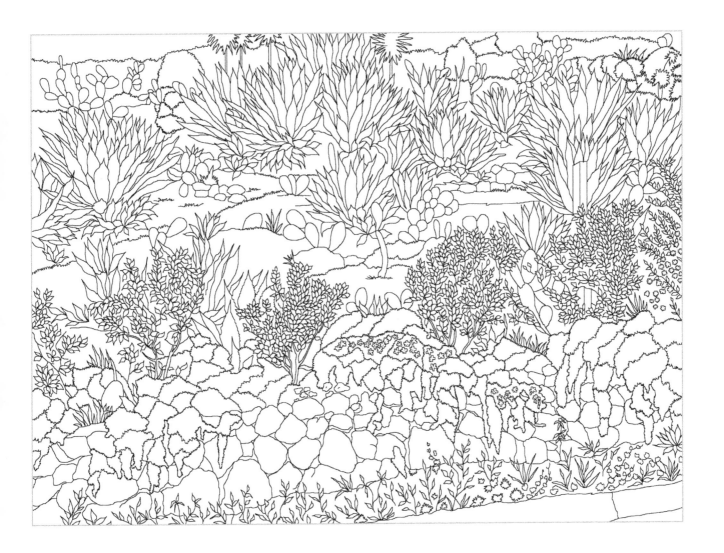

Brain resilience can be trained.

KEY TAKEAWAY:

Take a deep breath and then trace.

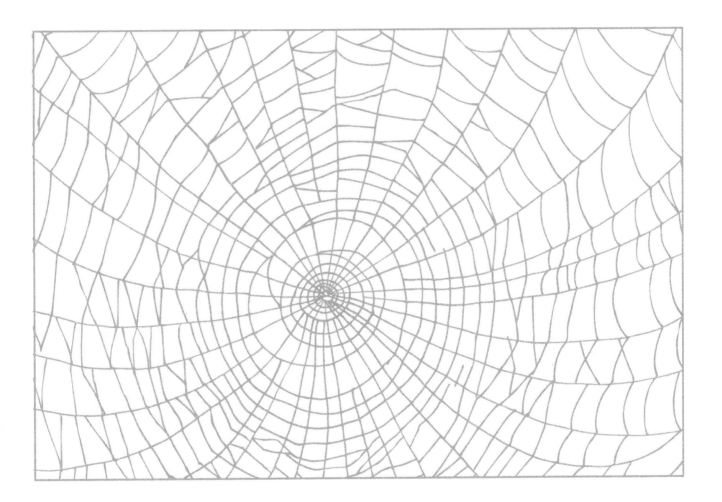

Clear the cobs of the past that keep the brain locked.

Train the brain. Change the future.

It starts by teaching the brain a new trick. Tracing instead of reacting to the situation. MiGGi prioritizes fear and stress over love and happiness to keep us feeling safe. It takes daily practice and time to rewire MiGGi.

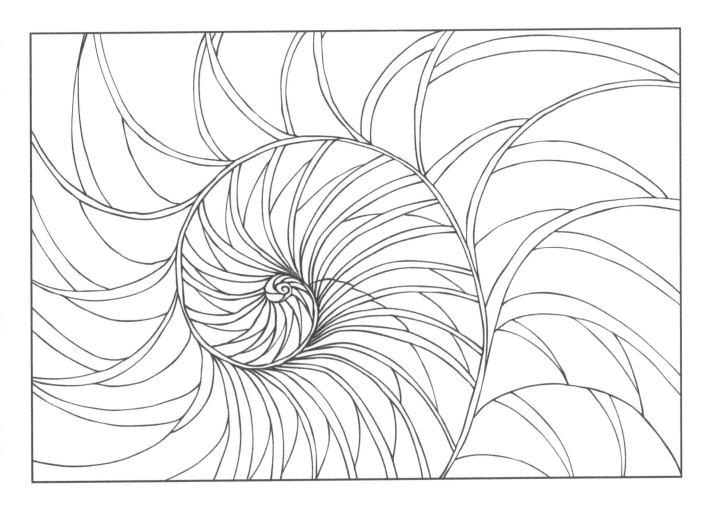

Reset your brain every morning as soon as you wake.

KEY TAKEAWAY:

Let It Go!

Write here what was going through your mind while tracing then let it go. This is a way to train the ancient part of the brain or (MiGGi) to not react. The repeated practice turns MiGGi reactions to Thinker responses. Then you learn a new way to respond to stressful or emotional situations.

_____

_____

_____

_____

_____

_____

_____

_____

_____

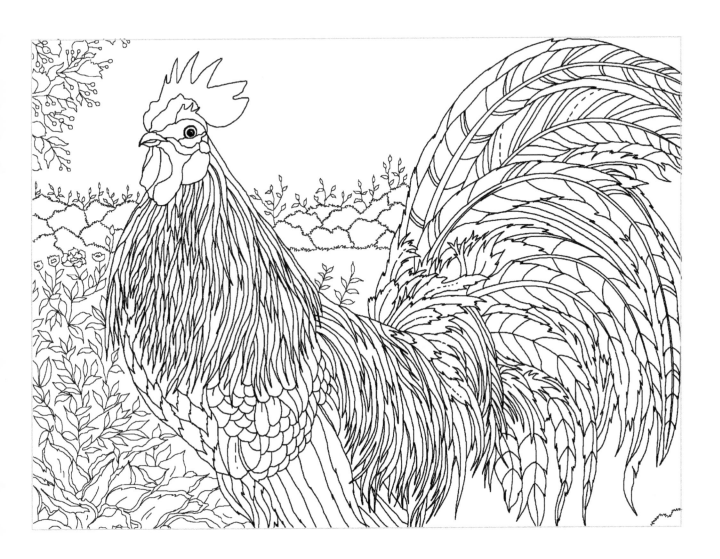

Switch off MiGGi. Switch on Thinker. Take charge of your brain.

KEY TAKEAWAY:

Train the brain like it is a muscle.

Trace it instead of react to it daily trains the brain to respond.

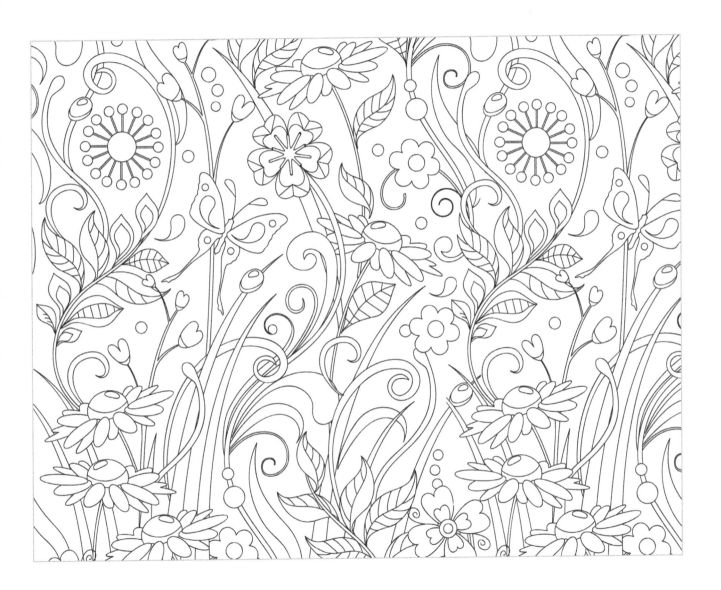

Prioritize nature over stress.

KEY TAKEAWAY:

You can teach an old dog new tricks!

Tracing everyday helps to retrain the brain to learn a healthier way to react to stressful situations. No matter what age.

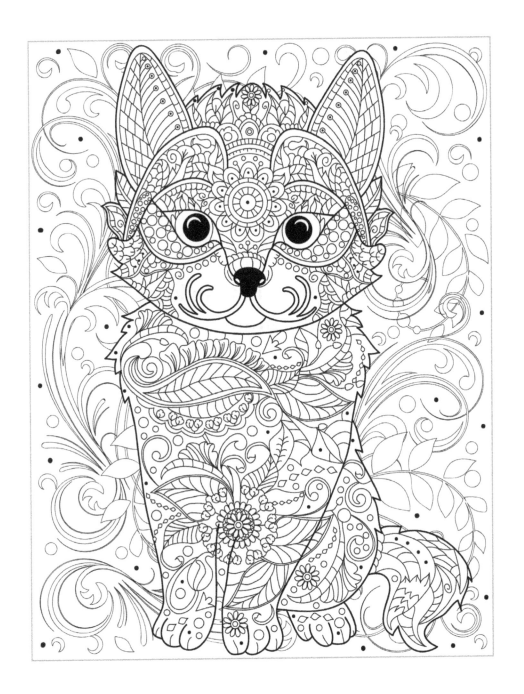

Never too late to start.

KEY TAKEAWAY:

There is nothing more powerful than knowing how to train the brain.

Just as you can learn to drive, or play tennis or speak another language, you can learn not to yell at someone or reach for that drink. Using the principles of neuroplasticity — the brain's ability to reorganize and change by forming new synapses, or neural connections, — you can retrain your brain.

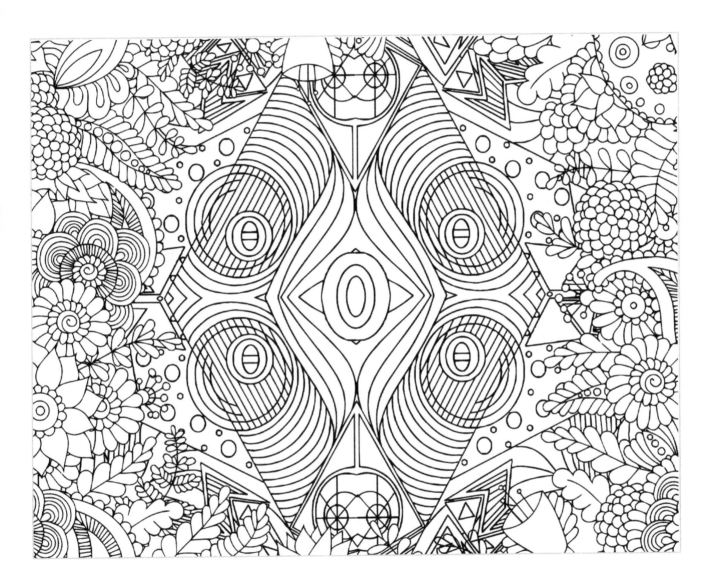

Unlock the beauty trapped inside MiGGi.

LEARN MORE ABOUT HOW TO GET A SMASHING MINDSET.

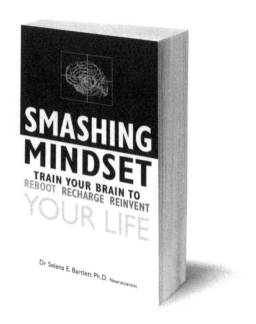

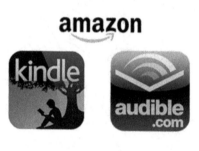

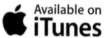

If you are interested in having Dr Selena Bartlett to host a speaking event or workshop please contact us at: info@smashmindset.com

For books, podcasts and to learn more about how to get a SMASHING MINDSET visit: www.selenab.com

Join our SMASHING MINDSET community on facebook at: facebook.com/smashing mindset

Follow us on Twitter: @traceiteraseit and Instagram: @1millionsmashingmindsets

CPSIA information can be obtained
at www.ICGtesting.com
Printed in the USA
LVHW061421120121
676304LV00036B/1001